Instant Pot Whole 30 Cookbook:

The Complete Whole 30 Instant Pot Cookbook - with 60 Healthy & Delicious Instant Pot Cooker Recipes

By Christine J. Coleman

© **Copyright 2017 by Christine J. Coleman - All rights reserved.**

Legal Notice:

The book is copyright protected. This is only for personal use. You cannot amend, distribute, sell, use, quote or paraphrase any part or the content within this book without the consent of the author.

Disclaimer Notice:

Please note the information contained within this document is for educational and entertainment purposes only. Every attempt has been made to provide accurate, up to date and reliable complete information. No warranties of any kind are expressed or implied. Readers acknowledge that the author is not engaging in the rendering of legal, financial, medical or professional advice. The content of this book has been derived from various sources. Please consult a licensed professional before attempting any techniques outlined in this book.

By reading this document, the reader agrees that under no circumstances are is the author responsible for any loses, direct or indirect, which are incurred as a result the use of information contained within this document, including, but not limited to, —errors, omissions, or inaccuracies.

Part One: Introduction...7

   The Prevalence of Obesity and Chronic Diseases of Lifestyle... 7

   The A, B, Cs of Whole30 Diet.. 10

   The Whole30 Diet Program Unchained....................... 11

   The Whole30 Diet Rules..13

   The Health Benefits of the Whole30 Diet —Give it Just 30 Days.. 14

   Introduction to Instant Pot... 17

   Why You Need an Instant Pot Miracle in Your Home 19

   Great Tips for Using Your Instant Pot......................... 20

PART TWO: THE WHOLE30 DIET RECIPES................23

   WHOLE 30 BREAKFAST RECIPES............................. 23

      Quinoa w/ Cherry Tomatoes, Garlic & Mushrooms 23

      Sausage, Leek & Asparagus Dill Breakfast Casserole 25

      Korean Steamed Breakfast Eggs................................ 27

      Breakfast Eggs de Provence....................................... 28

      Instant Pot Breakfast Casserole................................ 29

      Instant Pot Make-Ahead Detox Quinoa Breakfast Bowls.. 31

      Easy Breakfast Casserole... 32

      Tomato Dill Frittata.. 34

      Instant Pot Hot Breakfast Fruit Salad...................... 35

Instant Pot Egg & Ham Casserole.. 36
Instant Pot Tapioca Pudding.. 38
Instant Pot Buckwheat Porridge..39
Spicy Gluten-Free Pancakes..40
Hot Breakfast Bowl.. 42
Samoan Coconut Tapioca Porridge....................................43
Toast with Refried Beans and Avocado............................ 44

WHOLE 30 LUNCH RECIPES.. 46

Peperonata (Tasty Pepper Salad).. 46
Tasty Instant Pot Greek Fish Stew...................................... 47
Thai Red Curry with Kabocha Squash...............................49
Cream of Butternut Squash & Ginger Soup..................... 51
Tasty Mushroom Coconut Milk Soup................................ 52
Instant Pot Healthy Vegetable Stew...................................54
Mediterranean Quinoa Salad... 56
Instant Pot Ratatouille... 57
Instant Pot Detox Veggie Soup.. 59
Instant Pot Spicy Green Soup.. 60
Red Onion & Apple Soup.. 62
Mixed Veggie Noodles w/ Spicy Coconut Sauce..... 63
Sage-Infused Butternut Squash Zucchini Noodles.65
Instant Pot Coconut Cabbage...67
Yummy Brussels Sprouts... 68
Instant Pot Garlicky Mashed Potatoes............................... 70

INSTANT POT WHOLE30 DINNER RECIPES......... 71

Instant Pot Beef and Sweet Potato Stew.................... 71

Instant Pot Turkey Chili.. 73

Healthy Instant Pot Ground Beef Jalapeno Stew... 74

Instant Pot Italian Pulled Pork Ragu........................ 76

Jamaican Jerk Pork Roast – Low Carb & Whole 30 77

Instant Pot Barbacoa.. 78

Pressure Cooker AIP Italian Beef (Paleo, Gluten Free, Instant Pot)... 80

Healthy Quinoa Bowl with Grilled Steak & Veggies 81

Asparagus Quinoa & Steak Bowl............................. 83

Instant Pot Lemon Olive Chicken............................ 84

Instant Pot Chicken Shawarma................................ 86

Instant Pot Chipotle Shredded Beef........................ 87

Delicious Instant Pot Seafood Stew......................... 89

Instant Pot Coconut Curry Shrimp.......................... 90

Slow Cooker Thai Seafood Boil................................ 92

Hot Lemony Instant Pot Tilapia with Asparagus... 94

Instant Pot Citrus Tilapia.. 95

INSTANT POT WHOLE30 DESSERTS AND SNACKS 96

Power Protein Stuffed Strawberries........................ 96

Avocado Brownies.. 98

Instant Pot Blood Orange Marmalade................... 100

Instant Pot Cheesecake.. 101

Instant Pot Dulce de Leche..103
Ratatouille Riviera-Style...104
Lemon Broccoli..105
Instant Pot Baked Potatoes... 106
Strawberry-Rhubarb Compote w/ Fresh Mint......107
Parting Shot.. 109

Part One: Introduction

The Prevalence of Obesity and Chronic Diseases of Lifestyle

So many of us have poor eating habits without even knowing it; this could be attributed to an eating disorder, but often, it is purely disordered eating. Is it because we have come to rely on foods that are made in a plant instead of growing as a plant? One thing I know is that nature never intended for us to eat from a box that has been on a shelf somewhere for over two months, which most of us do. So, what do we expect when we defy nature? Weight gain and a host of diseases!

When walking down the street or going about your daily activities, what's the most prominent thing that catches your eye? For me, it's the rising number of overweight and obese people, and sadly, children have not been left behind. Consider the fact that all these you can see from the outside, but what about what's going on in the body you can't see with your naked eye?

The question to ask ourselves is, what happened? When and why did we suddenly become fat?

The answer is actually quite simple – the moment we started stuffing ourselves with processed food! There is a common phrase in technology that I really like to use in relation to health, and it goes, '**garbage in, garbage out**.' Taking it literally, if you feed your body with pure, healthy, natural, whole food, you are going to be in the epitome of health. If, on the other hand, you consistently feed on sweet, fatty, processed, and fast foods, I am sorry to say you are going to look and feel like junk.

It's important that you understand that eating junk, fast, and processed food is the precursor of the diseases of civilization, including obesity.

What does the ever-increasing number of overweight and obese people mean for our country and the world in general? There may come a time when life expectancy will be only 40 due to the rampancy of the diseases of civilization – obesity, diabetes, cancer, heart disease, and the like.

If nothing is done, we will no longer be productive people as most of us will be sick in hospitals or waiting to die in peace at home. Can you imagine how this would impact our economy, let alone our wellbeing?

Well, it's not all bad news. The whole foods diet is the embodiment of what nature intended for you to eat – fresh, natural, whole foods. But what does 'whole' really mean? It's not that you need to eat your food whole, rather it means eating food that still looks as it did growing as a plant, or very close to it, in short, food that has not been messed with through processing or only minimally messed with. Everything in that whole legume, fruit, nut, seed or veggie has already been perfectly arranged by nature, and as we know, **'don't mess with mother nature.'**

It is for this reason that I was inspired to write this book. I won't lie, embarking on the Whole 30 is no child's play, yet if you say this is hard, what will a person battling cancer say?

We are now going to get into the 30-day whole food program. Each chapter builds on the previous one with valuable tips that have helped many people lose weight, grow strong, and enjoy better health within just 30 days and a unique blend of yummy recipes.

All of the information you are about to read has been thoroughly researched by both leading scientists and the humble author to ensure that you get the best results you seek. So, let's get started on our mission to make you fit healthy and happy with life!

The A, B, Cs of Whole30 Diet

Think of the whole30 diet as pushing the 'reset' button for your overall health, relationship with food, and your habits.

Our premise is actually quite simple: the food you eat will affect your health either positively or negatively. There's no gray area, it's either black or white – every bite you take is either nourishing your body or making you fat and sick.

This makes everything so simple, right? You only eat the foods that are going to affect your life positively.

Hmmm. Actually, it partly is, and it partly isn't.

So many things come into play when it comes to making food choices and not just whether or not the food in question is healthy.

Have you ever wondered why, after a nasty breakup or a very bad day at work, you feel like drowning your sorrows in a whole tub of ice cream or a box of chocolates? This is because food is highly emotional, and sweet foods trigger the release of dopamine and serotonin, which are the feel-good hormones that can uplift your mood.

Food is also very sneaky; you could have just come back from lunch; then, on seeing a box of yummy looking donuts on your colleague's desk, you get an intense craving, like someone who hasn't eaten for a week!

As if this were not challenging enough to staying on the healthy track, every street corner today has a fast food joint, and if the hunger pangs hit you, convincing yourself to wait until you get home and have a healthy meal when all the French fries and burgers seem to be calling you by name can be quite an uphill task.

But wait, we are going to make it easy!

We will start by explaining the whole30 concept and all the benefits you stand to gain that are backed by scientific research. We will give you tasty recipes to help launch you into this program and conclusions that sum up the whole30 program. Then, we will set you out on a journey to recovering your health.

This program will turn you into an experimental guinea pig, so you can do some introspective work and figure yourself out. By the end of this program, you will have firsthand experience in the effects of healthy and natural foods and less healthy and processed foods.

All this in just 30 days!

The Whole30 Diet Program Unchained

As you get ready to embark on the Whole30 journey, the first thing you need to understand is that your health, weight, and overall wellbeing are determined by what you eat. Everything starts with food!

Certain food groups (such as processed foods, dairy, grains, sugar, and legumes) can have a negative effect on your overall health without you even noticing it. Do you have pains and aches that you can't explain? Are you always in need of recharging your batteries? Have you tried to lose weight with no success no matter how hard you try? Do you have a medical condition (such as fertility issues, digestive disorders, skin infections, etc.) for which medication doesn't seem to help?

These problems may be directly related to your diet, even what you might consider to be the 'healthy stuff.'

The challenge is to figure out if and how these foods are affecting you.

The solution is quite simple – strip them from your diet for a whole 30 days!

Cut out all the hormone unbalancing, inflammatory, and psychologically unhealthy and gut disrupting food groups for a month and give your body a fighting chance to recover and heal from the effects of these foods.

It's time to push the 'reset' button on your systemic inflammation, metabolism, and the downstream effects of the diet choices you've made.

It's time to learn, once and for all, how your food choices are affecting your daily life and your long-term health.

The Whole30 Diet Rules

- **Yes: eat natural and real food**

Eat tons of fresh vegetables, seafood, some fruit, meat, and plenty of good fats from seeds, fruits, nuts, fatty fish like salmon, and oils. Eat foods with few pronounceable ingredients or, better yet, foods with no listed ingredients because they are in their pure and natural form.

- **No: foods not to eat for 30 days**

Most importantly, here's what to AVOID for the 30 days. Omitting all these foods will help you regain your energy, healthy metabolism and significantly reduce systemic inflammation and help you discover how these foods have been affecting your health, quality of life, and fitness.

- Stay away from sugar of all kinds (artificial or natural)
- Don't consume any alcohol (not even in your cooking)
- Don't eat any grains or legumes
- Don't eat any dairy

- Don't take any MSG, carrageenan or sulfites (check your food labels)
- Don't try to recreate treats, baked foods or junk foods with the approved ingredients – continuing to eat your old and unhealthy foods made using whole 30 approved ingredients by, for example, making kale chips is totally missing the point. Remember, these are the same foods that got you into the trouble you are in with your health.

One final rule: you should not take any body measurements or step on the scale for the 30-day duration, so you can focus on your whole self and not just the weight aspect.

Exceptions to the rule

The following foods are allowed for your whole 30.

- Fresh fruit juice as a sweetener
- Clarified butter or ghee
- Vinegar
- Certain legumes such as snow peas, green beans, and sugar snap peas because they are more 'pod' and green matter than 'grain.'
- Salt

The Health Benefits of the Whole30 Diet – Give it Just 30 Days

Your role during the whole30 is to focus on making healthy, natural food choices, without having to stress about grass-fed, organic, free-range or pasture. Simply, figure out how to stick to the 30-day whole food program in any setting, under any amount of stress, around every special circumstance... for 30 days straight. Your only job? Eating healthy food!

By doing this, you are going to:

1. Sleep like an angel

When sugar is out the window, and healthy protein and fats are in, you will sleep like a baby without tossing and turning at 2.00 a.m.

2. Enjoy full-blown and consistent energy

Forget about energy highs and lows like a rollercoaster ride; you are going to have so much energy the Energizer bunny will be no match for you.

3. Wake well rested and alert

No need for your morning coffee to give you a jolt. All your batteries will be recharged, and you will wake up with a smile and an open heart ready to take on the world.

4. Bid farewell to digestive distress

Forget about tummy rumbles and unending gas. You might have a little discomfort if your previous diet did not feature lots of veggies, but after that, it's smooth sailing all the way.

5. Be clear headed and focused

Forget about the tip-of-the-tongue syndrome and brain fog. You will be more alert than ever.

6. Know the difference between real hunger and emotional appetite

You are already familiar with the mindless eating linked to emotional stress. This is emotional appetite, and it's typically 'junky.' As the body gets rid of sugar and settles into proper insulin management, the appetite diminishes, and real hunger – the need for nutritious food – will signal you when to eat.

7. Find new favorite foods

There's so much room on your plate and in your kitchen for new tastes, now that all the junk is out, and who knows which spices, veggies, fruits, and meats will become your new favorites?

8. Discover the fountain of youth

Your hair will be shinier and healthier; your skin will be more supple and tighter, and you will have shed some of the extra pounds. You will love it!

These are just the tip of the iceberg. Give the program a try, and you will discover a whole world of benefits. You will never want to look back!

Introduction to Instant Pot

You are at a point in life when you know you need to make some healthy choices, especially when it comes to food. However, you don't seem to have a spare minute to cook a healthy meal when you get home from work. The result? Takeout that you are genuinely fed up with, but the mere thought of fighting with pans and pots in your kitchen is almost unbearable after a long day at work.

This is where our Instant Pot Recipes come in. This book will show you that it is possible to make the healthiest meals for your family without breaking a sweat. It's as easy as combining all the ingredients of your meal in your instant pot, and in a snap, you have a hot, tasty dish ready and waiting.

If this sounds too good to be true, well, we haven't even gotten to the best part! You can prepare and cook all your meals in advance, say, during the weekend or when you have some free time. Once your food is ready, let it cool and pack it in your freezer. Come weekdays, you take out the food, thaw it, and you have a delicious, home-cooked dinner. Forget about the frozen food from your supermarket; you can now make your own.

We will start by teaching you the basics of using an instant pot and why you need to have one if you don't already, health benefits of following a vegetarian diet, and, lastly, healthy vegetarian recipes that you can make for your family, stress free.

Now, get your reading glasses, put your apron on standby, and let's get into this cooking adventure!

Why You Need an Instant Pot Miracle in Your Home

Have you ever dreamt of making a tasty and healthy meal in a snap, especially when you're in a hurry? Well, the instant pot is the surest way to make your dream come true! Forget about running around like a headless chicken trying to find the right ingredients and whipping them up together to make a decent meal for dinner when you can barely stay upright because of how tired you are. We are talking about throwing all the ingredients in one cooker to make the yummiest, well done meal in minutes!

Here are some more benefits of cooking using an instant pot that will have you going out to buy one immediately if you don't already have one.

- **Delicious and nutritious dishes**

Usually, meats and fresh vegetables are cooked in an instant pot for a few minutes, at a high temperature. As a result, nutrition-packed juices from the meats and veggies are released and retained as there is no escape through steam, meaning you get the best of flavors and nutrients.

- **Saves a lot of your time**

Perhaps the most attractive thing about using an instant pot is that you are not going crazy in the kitchen over a pot of food, checking it every few minutes so it doesn't burn. The only thing you may have to do with this cooker, especially if you are cooking meat, is to brown it in some oil over a stove top, if you want to have some great color in your stew; then, throw all the ingredients in your pot and come back to it once the cooking time is over.

- **Timeless**

An instant pot is a piece of kitchen equipment you can use all year round for many years to come and is not just limited to hot bowls of soup and stews for winter. You can use it to make yummy desserts and casseroles to be enjoyed during the summer, the beauty being you can use it in place of the oven so you don't make an already sweltering kitchen hotter. Better still, you can leave a casserole or meal of choice cooked before you go have fun at the beach, or somewhere else cooler; then, come back to a ready meal.

- **Easy to freeze**

Most meals cooked in an instant pot can be packed and stored in your freezer to be eaten at a later date, saving you even more time.

Great Tips for Using Your Instant Pot

- **Prep in advance**

If your mornings are busy, prepare everything you will need for your meal the night before. When using an instant pot, your ingredients should ideally be at room temperature or as close to it as possible. So, you can take out your ingredients from the fridge, immediately you get up in the morning, and let them warm up for about 20-30 minutes before turning on your pot. Cook your meals in minutes before leaving. You'll come back to a healthy meal in the evening.

- **Trim excess fat**

The beauty of using an instant pot is you don't need to add oil to your meals, especially if they are meat based. They won't stick to the bottom as long as there is enough moisture in the pot. Usually, when you cook meat on the stove top, the fat tends to drain away on its own but this is not the case in an instant pot and if you don't trim off the excess fat, you may end up with pools of oil in your stew.

For a tastier and healthier result, trim off excess fat.

- **Go easy on the soup**

When cooking using an instant pot, the moisture doesn't evaporate since it cooks with a tightly sealed lid throughout. When adapting a recipe that's typically cooked on a stove top, it's advisable to reduce the liquid content by about a third. As a rule of thumb, the soup/liquid should only just cover the ingredients. Otherwise, overfilling your pot with soup or liquid may lead to a leakage from the top and risk your food not cooking as well as it should.

When filling your pot with ingredients, don't go past the three quarter-way mark.

- **Thickening your sauce**

The fact that soup doesn't easily reduce in an instant pot means that it also doesn't thicken. If you like your broth or sauces nice and thick, you can roll your meat chunks in flour before browning them and adding them to the pot or alternatively, you can add a bit of cornstarch-water mixture towards the end of your cooking. Add it within the last five minutes of cooking time.

- **Don't be a peeping Tom**

Instant pots are designed to do their own thing. All you do is add your ingredients, seal the lid, turn it on and leave it to cook for the required period. If you are constantly checking the progress of your meal, you will have to increase the cooking time because every time you remove the lid, you release some heat. Needless to say, it's very dangerous to open the pot while the pressure is high, and your meal won't be as glorious as it would have been had you trusted the instant pot to do its thing!

- **When to add ingredients**

The best instant pot recipes, like the ones we are going to share in our next section, are those in which most of the ingredients are added at the beginning of the cooking process. This leaves you with a lot of time to do other things.

PART TWO: THE WHOLE30 DIET RECIPES

WHOLE 30 BREAKFAST RECIPES

Quinoa w/ Cherry Tomatoes, Garlic & Mushrooms

Yield: 3 Servings

Total Time: 17 Minutes

Prep Time: 7 Minutes

Cook Time: 10 Minutes

Ingredients

- 1 cup quinoa
- 3 tbsp. extra-virgin olive oil
- 4 cloves garlic, diced
- 15 medium button mushrooms, sliced
- 2 tbsp. fresh lemon juice
- 1 tbsp. lemon zest
- 1 red onion, diced
- 1 medium carrot, diced
- 8-10 cherry tomatoes
- 1 cup vegetable stock
- 1 tsp. sea salt
- Pinch of ground pepper

- Chopped spring onion and parsley to garnish

Directions

Press sauté button on your instant pot and heat the oil; stir in carrot and onion and cook for about 2 minutes. Stir in mushrooms for about 4 minutes and then stir in garlic, mushrooms, pepper, lemon juice and zest. Press cancel of warm button to stop cooking.

Stir in quinoa and then add cherry tomatoes; lock the lid and press the manual, high pressure button for 10 minutes. Natural release pressure and serve quinoa garnished with chopped spring onion and fresh herbs.

Nutritional Information per Serving:

Calories: 442; Total Fat: 18.5 g; Carbs: 59.8 g; Dietary Fiber: 10.5 g; Sugars: 13.3 g; Protein: 14.8 g; Cholesterol: 0 mg; Sodium: 683 mg

Sausage, Leek & Asparagus Dill Breakfast Casserole

Yields: 4 to 6 Servings

Total Time: 50 Minutes

Prep Time: 10 Minutes

Cook Time: 25 Minutes

Ingredients

- Coconut oil, for greasing the dish
- 1 pound breakfast sausage
- ¼ cup coconut milk
- 8 free range eggs, beaten
- ½ cup coconut cream
- 1 tbsp. minced fresh dill
- 6-8 stalks asparagus, chopped
- 1 thinly sliced leek
- ¼ tsp. garlic powder
- Sea salt and pepper

Directions

Grease a square baking dish and set aside.

Place the sausages in a pan set over medium heat; break them into small pieces. Cook for a few minutes and add asparagus and leeks; continue cooking for about 5 minutes more or until sausage is no longer pink. Remove the pan from heat, discarding excess fat.

Whisk together eggs, garlic powder, dill, cream, salt and pepper in a bowl; pour the mixture into the prepared baking dish and add the sausage mixture; mix well. Add water to the instant pot and insert a trivet; place the dish onto the trivet and lock lid. Cook on high for 25 minutes and then let pressure release on its own. Remove the casserole and cut into equal slices.

Nutritional Information per Serving:

Calories: 442; Total Fat: 18.5 g; Carbs: 59.8 g; Dietary Fiber: 10.5 g; Sugars: 13.3 g; Protein: 14.8 g; Cholesterol: 0 mg; Sodium: 683 mg

Korean Steamed Breakfast Eggs

Yield: 1 Serving

Total time: 10 Minutes

Prep time: 5 Minutes

Cook time: 5 Minutes

Ingredients

- 1 large egg
- pinch of sesame seeds
- 1 tsp. chopped scallions
- 1/3 cup cold water
- pinch of garlic powder
- pinch of salt
- pinch of pepper

Directions

In a small bowl, whisk together water and eggs until frothy; strain the mixture through a fine mesh into a heatproof bowl. Whisk in the remaining ingredients until well combined; set aside.

Add a cup of water to an instant pot and place a steamer basket or trivet in the pot; place the bowl with the mixture over the basket and lock lid. Cook on high for 5 minutes and then naturally release pressure.

Serve hot with a glass of freshly squeezed orange juice.

Nutritional Information per Serving:

Calories: 76; Total Fat: 5.2 g; Carbs: 0.9 g; Dietary Fiber: 0.2 g; Sugars: 0.5 g; Protein: 6.5 g; Cholesterol: 186 mg; Sodium: 228 mg

Breakfast Eggs de Provence

Yield: 6 Servings

Total time: 40 Minutes

Prep time: 10 Minutes

Cook time: 30 Minutes

Ingredients

- 1/2 cup coconut cream
- 6 eggs
- 1 cup cooked ham
- 1 red onion, chopped
- 1 cup vegan cheddar cheese
- 1 cup chopped kale leaves
- 1 tsp. Herbes de Provence
- 1/8 tsp. sea salt
- 1/8 tsp. pepper

Directions

In a bowl, whisk together coconut cream and eggs until well combined; stir in the remaining ingredients and pour the mixture into a heatproof bowl or dish; cover.

Add a cup of water to your instant pot and place a trivet over water. Add the bowl and lock lid; cook on high for 20 minutes and then release pressure naturally. Serve hot with a glass of fresh orange juice.

Nutritional Information per Serving:

Calories: 285; Total Fat: 18.3 g; Carbs: 14.4 g; Dietary Fiber: 5 g; Sugars: 2.6 g; Protein: 16.6 g; Cholesterol: 177 mg; Sodium: 561 mg

Instant Pot Breakfast Casserole

Yield: 6 Servings

Total Time: 45 Minutes

Prep Time: 15 Minutes

Cook Time: 30 Minutes

Ingredients

- 2 tbsp. coconut oil

- 1 ⅓ cups sliced leek
- 2 tsp. minced garlic
- 1 cup chopped kale
- 8 eggs
- ⅔ cups sweet potato, peeled and grated
- 1 ½ cups breakfast sausage

Directions

Set your instant pot to sauté mode and heat coconut oil; stir in garlic, leeks, and kale and sauté for about 5 minutes or until tender; transfer the veggies to a plate and clean the pot.

Whisk together eggs, beef sausage, sweet potato and the sautéed veggies in a large bowl until well blended; pour the mixture in a heatproof bowl or pan. Add water to the instant pot and insert a trivet; place the bowl onto the trivet and lock lid. Cook on manual for 25 minutes and then let pressure come down on its own. Remove the casserole and cut into equal slices.

Nutritional Information per Serving:

Calories: 280; Total Fat: 19 g; Carbs: 7 g; Dietary Fiber: 1 g; Sugars: 2 g; Protein: 25 g; Cholesterol: 295 mg; Sodium: 160 mg

Instant Pot Make-Ahead Detox Quinoa Breakfast Bowls

Yield: 4 Servings

Total Time: 26 Minutes

Prep Time: 25 Minutes

Cook Time: 1 Minute

Ingredients

Quinoa:

- 2 cups coconut milk
- 1 1/2 cups water
- 1 1/2 cups quinoa, soaked for at least 1 hour, drained and rinsed
- 2 tsp. vanilla extract
- 1/4 cup raw honey
- 1 tsp. ground cinnamon
- 1/4 tsp. salt

Optional toppings:

- Coconut flakes
- Fresh fruit

Directions

Add quinoa to your instant pot and add in water, milk, vanilla, honey, cinnamon and salt; lock the lid and press the "rice" button.

When done, let pressure come down naturally and then divide the cooked quinoa into six serving bowls. Serve topped with coconut flakes and fresh fruit. Enjoy!

Nutritional Information per Serving:

Calories: 712; Total Fat: 46.9 g; Carbs: 65.6 g; Dietary Fiber: 9.3 g; Sugars: 18.2 g; Protein: 13.2 g; Cholesterol: 0 mg; Sodium: 182 mg

Easy Breakfast Casserole

Yields: 5 to 6 Servings

Total Time: 50 Minutes

Prep Time: 25 Minutes

Cook Time: 25 Minutes

Ingredients

- 1½ pound breakfast sausage
- 1 large yam or sweet potato, diced
- 2 tbsp. melted coconut oil
- 10 eggs, whisked
- ½ tsp. garlic powder
- 2 cups chopped spinach
- ½ yellow onion, diced
- ½ tsp. sea salt

Directions

Coat a 9x12 baking dish with cooking spray.

Toss the diced sweet potatoes in coconut oil and sprinkle with salt. Set aside.

Set a sauté pan over medium heat; add yellow onion and sauté for about 4 minutes or until fragrant. Stir in breakfast sausage and cook for about 5 minutes or until the sausages are no longer pink.

Transfer the sausage mixture to the baking dish and add spinach and sweet potatoes. Top with eggs and sprinkle with garlic powder and salt. Mix until well combined and pour the mixture in a heatproof bowl or pan. Add water to the instant pot and insert a trivet; place the dish on the trivet and lock the lid. Cook on high for 25 minutes and then let pressure come down on its own. Remove the casserole and cut into equal slices.

Nutritional Information per Serving:

Calories: 76; Total Fat: 5.2 g; Carbs: 0.9 g; Dietary Fiber: 0.2 g; Sugars: 0.5 g; Protein: 6.5 g; Cholesterol: 186 mg; Sodium: 228 mg

Tomato Dill Frittata

Yields: 4 Servings

Total Time: 30 Minutes

Prep Time: 10 Minutes

Cook Time: 20 Minutes

Ingredients

- 8 free-range eggs, whisked
- 2 tbsp. chopped fresh chives
- 2 tbsp. chopped fresh dill
- 4 tomatoes, diced
- 1 tsp. red pepper flakes
- 2 garlic cloves, minced
- Coconut oil, for greasing the pan
- Sea salt
- Black pepper

Directions

Grease a cast iron skillet or saucepan and set aside.

In a large bowl, whisk together the eggs; beat in the remaining ingredients until well mixed.

Pour the egg mixture into the prepared pan and pour the mixture in a heatproof bowl or pan. Add water to the instant pot and insert a trivet; place the pan on the trivet and lock the lid. Cook on high for 20 minutes and then let pressure come down on its own. Remove the casserole and cut into equal slices.

Garnish the frittata with extra chives and dill to serve.

Nutritional Information per Serving:

Calories: 166; Total Fat: 10.3 g; Carbs: 7.2 g; Dietary Fiber: 1.9 g; Sugars: 4 g; Protein: 12.7 g; Cholesterol: 327 mg; Sodium: 250 mg

Instant Pot Hot Breakfast Fruit Salad

Yield: 10 Servings

Total Time: 25 Minutes

Prep Time: 10 Minutes

Cook Time: 15 Minutes

Ingredients

- 8 cups chopped pears
- 8 cups chopped peaches
- 1/2 cup coconut oil, melted
- 1/4 cup dried cranberries
- 1/2 cup dried apricots, chopped
- 3 cups chunky applesauce
- 1/4 tsp. ground nutmeg

- 1/4 tsp. ground cinnamon
- 3/4 cups raw honey
- 1/8 tsp. salt

Directions

Combine all ingredients in an instant pot and lock lid; press manual for 15 minutes. When done, quickly release the pressure and then serve.

Nutritional Information per Serving:

Calories: 330; Total Fat: 11.5 g; Carbs: 61.2 g; Dietary Fiber: 7.1 g; Sugars: 52.9 g; Protein: 1.9 g; Cholesterol: 0 mg; Sodium: 35 mg

Instant Pot Egg & Ham Casserole

Yield: 4 Servings

Total Time: 35 Minutes

Prep Time: 10 Minutes

Cook Time: 25 Minutes

Ingredients

- 1 cup almond milk
- 10 large eggs
- 2 cups shredded vegan cheddar cheese

- 1 cup chopped ham
- 1/2 onion, diced
- 4 medium red potatoes, chopped
- 1 tsp. salt
- 1 tsp. pepper

Directions

Grease an instant pot with nonstick cooking spray and add two cups of water; insert a steamer basket. Whisk almond milk and eggs in a bowl until well blended; mix in cheese, onion, ham, potatoes, salt and pepper until well combined. Transfer the egg mixture into a heatproof bowl and insert into the pot. Lock lid and press manual button; set for 25 minutes. When done, let pressure come down on its own and then serve the Casserole with your favorite toppings.

Nutritional Information per Serving:

Calories: 528; Total Fat: 30 g; Carbs: 41.1 g; Dietary Fiber: 5.8 g; Sugars: 5.7 g; Protein: 26.9 g; Cholesterol: 484 mg; Sodium: 1219 mg

Instant Pot Tapioca Pudding

Yield: 4-6 Servings

Total Time: 13 Minutes

Prep Time: 5 Minutes

Cook Time: 8 Minutes

Ingredients

- ⅓ cup seed tapioca pearls, rinsed
- 1¼ cups low-fat milk
- 1 tsp. lemon zest
- 2 tbsp. raw honey
- ½ cup water

Directions

Add water to your instant pot and insert a steamer basket. In a heat-proof bowl, whisk together milk, water, tapioca, honey, and lemon zest until well combined. Place the bowl into the pot and lock the lid. Cook on high pressure for eight minutes and then release the pressure naturally. Remove the bowl and stir the pudding before serving.

Serve topped with fruit.

Nutritional Information per Serving:

Calories: 187; Total Fat: 2.5 g; Carbs: 39.6 g; Dietary Fiber: 0.1 g; Sugars: 28.9 g; Protein: 2.5 g; Cholesterol: 7 mg; Sodium: 40 mg

Instant Pot Buckwheat Porridge

Yield: 3-4 Servings

Total time: 16 Minutes

Prep time: 10 Minutes

Cook time: 6 Minutes

Ingredients

- 1 cup raw buckwheat groats, rinsed
- 1 banana, sliced
- ¼ cup raisins
- 3 cups milk
- 1 tsp. ground cinnamon
- ½ tsp. vanilla
- chopped nuts

Directions

Add buckwheat to your instant pot and add raisins, banana, milk, vanilla, and cinnamon; lock lid and cook on high for six minutes. Let the pressure come down naturally.

Stir the porridge and serve topped with chopped nuts. Enjoy!

Nutritional Information per Serving:

Calories: 360; Total Fat: 16.2 g; Carbs: 50.4 g; Dietary Fiber: 6 g; Sugars: 9.1 g; Protein: 8.5 g; Cholesterol: 0 mg; Sodium: 239 mg

Spicy Gluten-Free Pancakes

Yield: 4 Servings

Total Time: 26 Minutes

Prep Time: 10 Minutes

Cook Time: 16 Minutes

Ingredients

- 4 tbsp. coconut oil
- 1 cup coconut milk
- ½ cup tapioca flour
- ½ cup almond flour
- 1 tsp. salt

- ½ tsp. chili powder
- ¼ tsp. turmeric powder
- ¼ tsp. black pepper
- ½ inch ginger, grated
- 1 serrano pepper, minced
- 1 handful cilantro, chopped
- ½ red onion, chopped

Directions

In a bowl, combine coconut milk, tapioca flour, almond flour, and spices until well blended; stir in ginger, Serrano pepper, cilantro, and red onion until well combined.

Grease the interior of the instant pot with coconut oil; pour in the batter and seal the pot with vent closed; set pressure to low and cook for 30 minutes.
Serve the crispy pancakes with freshly squeezed orange juice.

Nutritional Information per Serving:

Calories: 447; Total Fat: 34.6 g; Carbs: 34 g; Dietary Fiber: 3.3 g; Sugars: 2.7 g; Protein: 4.6 g; Cholesterol: 0 mg; Sodium: 600 mg

Hot Breakfast Bowl

Yield: 3 Servings

Total Time: 30 Minutes

Prep Time: 10 Minutes

Cook Time: 20 Minutes

Ingredients

- 2 cups quinoa
- 1 tbsp. coconut oil
- ¼ cup sunflower seeds
- ½ cup walnuts
- 1 cup fresh cranberries
- ½ tsp. cinnamon
- Raw honey to serve

Directions

Preheat oven to 400°F. Cook quinoa in an instant pot until tender. In a bowl, mix together coconut oil, sunflower seeds, walnuts, cranberries, and cinnamon until well blended. Transfer the mixture to a baking dish lined with parchment paper. Bake for about 20 minutes. Scoop out ¾ cup of the hot berry mixture over the cooked quinoa and drizzle with honey. Enjoy!

Nutritional Information per Serving:

Calories: 628; Total Fat: 25.7 g; Carbs: 79.2 g; Dietary Fiber: 11.2 g; Sugars: 1.7 g; Protein: 21.8 g; Cholesterol: 0 mg; Sodium: 7 mg

Samoan Coconut Tapioca Porridge

Yield: 2 Servings
Total Time: 15 Minutes
Prep Time: 10 Minutes
Cook Time: 5 Minutes

Ingredients:

- 1/4 cup tapioca
- 1 can coconut milk
- 1/3 cup raw honey
- 1 1/2 tsp. lemon juice
- 1/2 cup toasted coconut flakes

Directions

Soak tapioca in 2 cups of water in an instant pot for about 15 minutes; add honey and milk and lock the lid; cook on high pressure 5 minutes. Turn off your pot and release pressure naturally before opening the lid. The tapioca should be cooked through and translucent.

Stir in lemon juice and garnish with coconut flakes to serve.

Nutritional Information per Serving:

Calories: 541; Total Fat: 35.3 g; Carbs: 60 g; Dietary Fiber: 4.6 g; Sugars: 39.3 g; Protein: 3.5 g; Cholesterol: 0 mg; Sodium: 23 mg

Toast with Refried Beans and Avocado

Yield: 1 Serving

Total time: 35 Minutes

Prep Time: 15 Minutes

Cook Time: 20 Minutes

Ingredients

- 2 slices gluten-free bread
- 1 cup dry beans
- 1 avocado, thinly sliced
- Slivered white onion
- Sea salt

Directions

Soak the cup of beans in cold water for 6-8 hours and then boil in your instant pot for 20 minutes after attaining high pressure.

Turn off your instant pot and release pressure naturally for about 10 minutes and release any that's left manually, being very carefully not to get burnt by the steam.

Fry the beans and put them in your refrigerator.

When you are ready to make the sandwich, re-fry the beans and add any of your favorite herbs and spices.

Toast the bread to your liking. Top with the refried beans and avocado slices; scatter with silvered onions and sprinkle with salt to serve. Enjoy!

Nutritional Information per Serving:

Calories: 492; Total Fat: 39.9 g; Carbs: 34.2 g; Dietary Fiber: 17.6 g; Sugars: 3.3 g; Protein: 7.2 g; Cholesterol: 0 mg; Sodium: 141 mg

WHOLE 30 LUNCH RECIPES

Peperonata (Tasty Pepper Salad)

Yield: 4 Servings

Total Time: 15 Minutes

Prep Time: 5 Minutes

Cook Time: 10 Minutes

Ingredients:

- 2 red capsicums, sliced into strips
- 2 yellow capsicums, sliced into strips
- 1 green capsicum, sliced into strips
- ½ tsp. olive oil
- 1 red onion
- 2 garlic cloves
- 3 tomatoes, chopped
- basil, chopped
- salt and pepper

Directions

Add oil to your instant pot and sauté onions until tender; add one garlic clove and capsicums and cook until browned. Add the chopped tomatoes, salt, and pepper and stir to mix; lock lid and cook on high pressure for five minutes and then release pressure naturally.

Press the remaining garlic clove and set aside.

Remove capsicums into a bowl and add olive oil, garlic and chopped basil; mix well and serve.

Nutritional Information per Serving:

Calories: 48; Total Fat: 1.1 g; Carbs: 9.2 g; Dietary Fiber: 2.9 g; Sugars: 5.1 g; Protein: 1.8 g; Cholesterol: 0 mg; Sodium: 6 mg

Tasty Instant Pot Greek Fish Stew

Yield: 5 Servings

Total Time: 30 Minutes

Prep Time: 10 Minutes

Cook Time: 20 Minutes

Ingredients

- 5 large white fish fillets
- 1 large red onion, chopped
- 4 cloves of garlic
- 1 leek, sliced
- 1 carrot, chopped
- 3 sticks celery, chopped
- 1 can tomatoes

- 1/2 tsp. saffron threads
- 8 cups fish stock
- 2 tbsp. fresh lemon juice
- 1 tbsp. lemon zest
- handful parsley leaves chopped
- handful mint leaves chopped

Directions

Combine all ingredients in your instant pot and lock lid; cook on high for 20 minutes and then release pressure naturally. Serve with gluten-free bread.

Nutritional Information per Serving:

Calories: 443; Total Fat: 18.4 g; Carbs: 9.7 g; Dietary Fiber: 1.8 g; Sugars: 3.5 g; Protein: 58.8 g; Cholesterol: 153 mg; Sodium: 871 mg

Thai Red Curry with Kabocha Squash

Yield: 4-6 Servings

Total Time: 30 Minutes

Prep Time: 10 Minutes

Cook Time: 20 Minutes

Ingredients

- 3 pounds squash, peeled, seeded, and diced
- 1 tbsp. vegetable oil
- 1 medium red onion, diced
- 1 tbsp. ginger, grated
- 4 medium garlic cloves, chopped
- 2 medium green bell peppers, cut into 1/4-inch strips
- 1 1/2 tsp. salt
- 1/2 cup water
- 2 cups coconut milk
- 3 tbsp. Thai red curry paste
- 1 tbsp. soy sauce
- 1/4 cup chopped cilantro
- 2 tsp. freshly squeezed lime juice
- Steamed cooked quinoa, for serving

Directions

In a large pan, heat oil until hot but not smoking; stir in onion and a tsp. of salt; cook for about 6 minutes or until onion is tender. Stir in ginger, garlic, and peppers and cook for one minute more or until fragrant.

Transfer to your instant pot and stir in the remaining ingredients except lime juice and cilantro. Lock lid and cook on high for 20 minutes. Release pressure naturally and then stir in lime juice and cilantro; serve hot over cooked quinoa.

Nutritional Information per Serving:

Calories: 399; Total Fat: 1.1 g; Carbs: 37.3 g; Dietary Fiber: 7.3 g; Sugars: 9.5 g; Protein: 9.4 g; Cholesterol: 0 mg; Sodium: 1161 mg

Cream of Butternut Squash & Ginger Soup

Yield: 4 Servings

Total Time: 25 Minutes

Prep Time: 5 Minutes

Cook Time: 20 Minutes

Ingredients

- 1 tsp. extra-virgin olive oil
- 1 large onion, roughly chopped
- 1 sprig of Sage
- 4 pound butternut Squash, diced
- ½" piece of fresh ginger, minced
- ¼ tsp. nutmeg
- salt and pepper
- 4 cups vegetable stock
- ½ cup toasted salted pumpkin seeds, to serve

Directions

In your instant pot, sauté onion with salt, pepper, and sage until softened. Remove the onion mixture to a bowl and add squash cubes to the pot; sauté for 10 minutes and then add in the remaining ingredients, including the onion mixture. Lock lid and cook on high pressure for 15 minutes; release pressure naturally and then discard sage. Using an immersion blender, blend the mixture until smooth and serve garnished with toasted pumpkin seeds.

Nutritional Information per Serving:

Calories: 323; Total Fat: 9.6 g; Carbs: 59.7 g; Dietary Fiber: 10.6 g; Sugars: 11.8 g; Protein: 9.2 g; Cholesterol: 0 mg; Sodium: 23 mg

Tasty Mushroom Coconut Milk Soup

Yield: 4 Servings

Total Time: 20 Minutes

Prep Time: 10 Minutes

Cook Time: 10 Minutes

Ingredients

- 1 ½ pounds mushroom, trimmed
- 1 clove garlic, minced
- 2 red onions, chopped
- 4 cups vegetable stock
- 2 cups coconut milk
- 1 tbsp. fresh thyme

- 1/8 tsp. sea salt
- Thyme sprigs
- 1/8 tsp. pepper

Directions

Grill the mushrooms, turning frequently, for about five minutes or until charred and tender; set aside.

In an instant pot, sauté red onion in a splash of water. Stir in vegetable stock and cook for a few minutes. Add the remaining ingredients and lock the lid; cook on high pressure for three minutes and then release the pressure naturally. Transfer the mixture to a blender and blend until very smooth. Serve garnished with thyme sprigs.

Nutritional Information per Serving:

Calories: 338; Total Fat: 29.2 g; Carbs: 18.1 g; Dietary Fiber: 5.8 g; Sugars: 9.3 g; Protein: 8.8 g; Cholesterol: 0 mg; Sodium: 89 mg

Instant Pot Healthy Vegetable Stew

Yield: 8 Servings

Total Time: 45 Minutes

Prep Time: 30 Minutes

Cook Time: 15 Minutes

Ingredients

- 1 cup Portobello mushrooms, chopped
- 1 cup white button mushrooms
- 1/4 cup vegetable broth
- 2 cloves garlic, minced
- 1 med carrot, minced
- 1 stalk celery, minced
- 1/2 med onion, minced
- 2 med Yukon gold potatoes, diced
- 1 cup green beans, cubed
- ½ cup frozen peas
- 1 stalk celery, chopped
- 2 medium carrots, chopped
- 2 tbsp. corn starch
- 3/4 cup pearl onions
- 1/2 tsp. rubbed sage
- 1 tsp. rosemary
- 3 cups vegetable broth
- 1 tbsp. balsamic vinegar
- 1 can tomato sauce

- 1 can diced tomatoes
- 1 tsp. Italian seasoning
- 1/2 tsp. sea salt
- 1/4 tsp. ground pepper

Directions

Set your instant pot to sauté mode and sauté garlic, onion, celery, and carrots for about four minutes; stir in sage, rosemary, and Italian seasoning for about 20 seconds. Stir in mushrooms and cook until all liquid is evaporated; deglaze with vinegar and stir in broth, tomato sauce, tomatoes, and the remaining veggies, except peas and pearl onion. Stir in seasoning and lock the lid; set on manual for 15 minutes. When done, natural release pressure; stir in peas, pearl onions, and starchy slurry. Serve.

Nutritional Information per Serving:

Calories: 154; Total Fat: 0.9 g; Carbs: 25.3 g; Dietary Fiber: 5.3 g; Sugars: 3.5 g; Protein: 11.9 g; Cholesterol: 0 mg; Sodium: 461 mg

Mediterranean Quinoa Salad

Yield: 2 Servings

Total Time: 20 Minutes
Prep Time: 10 Minutes
Cook Time: 10 Minutes

Ingredients

- 1 cup quinoa
- 4 black olives, pitted and chopped
- 3 slices bacon, cooked and chopped
- 2-4 cups mixed greens
- 2 tbsp. lemon juice
- ½ small cucumber, chopped
- 1 small tomato, diced
- 1 tbsp. red onion, chopped
- 1 tbsp. oregano
- Salt and pepper
- 4 tbsp. hummus

Directions

Cook quinoa in an instant pot until tender. Combine all the ingredients in a bowl, except hummus; cover with lid and shake well. Top with hummus and enjoy!

Nutritional Information per Serving:

Calories: 520; Total Fat: 9.6 g; Carbs: 89.7 g; Dietary Fiber: 18 g; Sugars: 8.8 g; Protein: 20.8 g; Cholesterol: 0 mg; Sodium: 258 mg

Instant Pot Ratatouille

Yield: 4 Servings
Total Time: 35 Minutes
Prep Time: 15 Minutes
Cook Time: 20 Minutes

Ingredients

- 1 eggplant, halved then sliced
- 1 green pepper, cut in strips (deseeded)
- 1 onion, halved then sliced
- 1 tomato, wedged
- 2 small zucchinis, sliced
- 75 ml tomato paste
- 1/8 cup olive oil
- 2 tbsp. fresh parsley
- 1 tsp. dried basil
- 1 tsp. sugar
- ½ tsp. oregano
- ½ tsp. freshly ground black pepper

- Salt and red pepper flakes to taste

Directions

Layer the vegetables in your instant pot, starting with onions, eggplant, zucchini, garlic, followed by the peppers and finally the tomatoes. Sprinkle with half the dried herbs, sugar, parsley, salt, and pepper flakes. Add half the tomato paste and repeat the layering in the same order.

Next, drizzle with the olive oil, lock lid, and cook on high pressure for 20 minutes. Release the pressure naturally and serve.

Nutritional Information per Serving:

Calories: 137; Total Fat: 6.9 g; Carbs: 19.1 g; Dietary Fiber: 7.2 g; Sugars: 10.7 g; Protein: 3.7 g; Cholesterol: 0 mg; Sodium: 33 mg

Instant Pot Detox Veggie Soup

Yield: 1 Serving
Total Time: 15 Minutes
Prep Time: 5 Minutes
Cook Time: 10 Minutes

Ingredients

- 1 medium cauliflower
- 8 cups water
- 1 tsp. lemon juice
- 3 tsp. ground flax seeds
- 3 cups spinach
- 1 tsp. cayenne pepper
- 1 tsp. black pepper
- 1 tsp. soy sauce

Directions:

Core cauliflower and cut the florets into large pieces; reserve stems for juicing.
Add cauliflower to an instant pot and add water; lock lid and cook on high pressure for 10 minutes. Release pressure naturally and transfer the cauliflower to a blender along with two cups of cooking liquid; blend

until very smooth. Add the remaining ingredients and continue blending until very smooth. Serve hot or warm.

Nutritional Information per Serving:

Calories: 198; Total Fat: 11.2 g; Carbs: 11.1 g; Dietary Fiber: 6.3 g; Sugars: 2.9 g; Protein: 1.8 g; Cholesterol: 0 mg; Sodium: 213 mg

Instant Pot Spicy Green Soup

Yield: 2 Servings
Total Time: 30 Minutes
Prep Time: 15 Minutes
Cook Time: 15 Minutes

Ingredients

- 5 cups water
- 1 cup chickpeas
- 1 green bell pepper, chopped
- 1 red onion, chopped
- 4 celery stalks, chopped
- 2 cups chopped spinach
- 1 tsp. dried mint
- 1/2 tsp. ground cumin

- 1/2 tsp. ground ginger
- 1/2 tsp. cardamom
- 2 cloves of garlic
- 1 tbsp. coconut milk
- Pinch of sea salt
- pinch of pepper

Directions:

Combine all ingredients, except spinach and coconut milk, in your instant pot and lock lid; cook on high pressure for 15 minutes and then release the pressure naturally. Stir in spinach; let sit for about 5 minutes and then blend the mixture until very smooth.

Serve the soup into soup bowls and add coconut milk. Season with salt and more pepper and enjoy!

Nutritional Information per Serving:

Calories: 317; Total Fat: 2.8 g; Carbs: 11.2 g; Dietary Fiber: 6.3 g; Sugars: 4 g; Protein: 12.3 g; Cholesterol: 0 mg; Sodium: 356 mg

Red Onion & Apple Soup

Yield: 6 Servings
Total Time: 25 Minutes
Prep Time: 10 Minutes
Cook Time: 15 Minutes

Ingredients

- 1 tbsp. canola oil
- 1 cup chopped red onion
- 3 organic apples, diced
- 8 cups vegetable broth
- 1/2 tbsp. chopped fresh rosemary
- 1 leek, chopped
- 1/2 tbsp. fresh thyme
- A pinch of cayenne pepper
- A pinch of sea salt

Directions

In a medium saucepan, heat canola oil; stir in onion and sauté for about four minutes or until fragrant and golden; transfer the sautéed onion to your instant pot, stir in broth, and bring the mixture to a gentle boil on sauté mode.

Stir in the apples, leek, thyme, and rosemary and lock lid; cook on high pressure for 10 minutes. When done, release pressure naturally; season with salt and pepper and serve.

Nutritional Information per Serving:

Calories: 342; Total Fat: 15.6 g; Carbs: 23.5 g; Dietary Fiber: 9.1 g; Sugars: 11.9 g; Protein: 1.2 g; Cholesterol: 0 mg; Sodium: 413 mg

Mixed Veggie Noodles w/ Spicy Coconut Sauce

Yield: 2 Servings

Total Time: 13 Minutes

Prep Time: 10 Minutes

Cook Time: 3 Minutes

Ingredients

- 2 green zucchinis
- 2 yellow zucchinis
- 7 ounces mangetout or fresh peas
- 2 corn cobs
- 1 handful of fresh mixed herbs, chopped

For the sauce:

- 1 banana shallot, chopped
- 2 tsp. ground turmeric
- 1 clove garlic, finely chopped
- 1 red chili, deseeded and chopped
- ½ tsp. ginger paste
- 10 ounces coconut water
- 7 ounces coconut milk
- 1 tsp. hot curry powder
- 4 ounces desiccated coconut, unsweetened
- Juice of 1 lime

Directions

Start by making the sauce.

Combine all the sauce ingredients in your food processor and pulse until perfectly smooth.

Using a spiralizer or julienne peeler, cut the carrot and zucchini into long, thin noodles. Combine with the rest of the veggies in a bowl. For the mangetout, slice it diagonally.

Add the veggies to a steam basket and insert into your instant pot with water and lock the lid. Cook on manual for three minutes and then let pressure come down on its own. Remove the basket from the pot and immediately transfer the veggies to a bowl. Serve the veggies drizzled with the spicy coconut sauce and garnished with the mixed herbs, cover and let marinate for half an hour.

Serve with lime wedges.

Nutritional Information per Serving:

Calories: 598; Total Fat: 36.2 g; Carbs: 53.4 g; Dietary Fiber: 16.8g; Sugars: 25.6 g; Protein: 18.8 g; Cholesterol: 28 mg; Sodium: 42 mg

Sage-Infused Butternut Squash Zucchini Noodles

Yield: 4 Servings

Total Time: 25 Minutes

Prep Time: 10 Minutes

Cook Time: 15 Minutes

Ingredients

- 3 large zucchinis, spiralized or julienned into noodles
- 3 cups cubed butternut squash
- 2 cloves garlic, finely chopped
- 1 yellow onion, chopped
- 2 tbsp. olive oil
- 2 cups homemade vegetable broth
- ¼ tsp. red pepper flakes
- Freshly ground black pepper
- 1 tbsp. fresh sage, finely chopped
- Salt, to taste and smoked salt for garnish

Directions

Add the oil to a pan over medium heat. Once it's hot, sauté the sage until crisp. Transfer to a small bowl, season lightly with salt, then set aside.

Add the onion, butternut, garlic, broth, salt, and pepper flakes to an instant pot and lock the lid; cook on high pressure for 10 minutes and then release pressure naturally.

Meanwhile, steam the zucchini noodles in your microwave or steamer until crisp-tender.

Once the butternut mixture is ready, remove from heat; let it cool off slightly, then transfer to a blender and process until smooth.

Combine the zucchini noodles and the butternut puree in the skillet over medium heat and cook until heated through and evenly coated for two minutes.

Sprinkle with fried sage and smoked salt and serve hot.

Nutritional Information per Serving:

Calories: 301; Total Fat: 28.5 g; Carbs: 13.8 g; Dietary Fiber: 3.4g; Sugars: 4.8 g; Protein: 1.9 g; Cholesterol: 0 mg; Sodium: 161 mg

Instant Pot Coconut Cabbage

Yield: 6-8 Servings

Total Time: 25 Minutes

Prep Time: 15 Minutes

Cook Time: 10 Minutes

Ingredients

- 1 tbsp. coconut oil
- 1 tbsp. olive oil
- ½ cup desiccated unsweetened coconut
- 2 tbsp. lemon juice
- 1 medium carrot, sliced
- 1 medium brown onion, sliced
- 1 medium cabbage, shredded
- 1 tbsp. turmeric powder
- 1 tbsp. mild curry powder
- 1 tsp. mustard powder
- ½ long red chili, sliced
- 2 large cloves of garlic, diced
- 1½ tsp. salt
- ⅓ cup water

Directions

Turn your instant pot on sauté mode and add coconut oil; stir in onion and salt and cook for about four minutes. Stir in spices, chili, and garlic for about 30 seconds. Stir in the remaining ingredients and lock the lid; set on manual high for five minutes. When done, natural release the pressure and stir the mixture. Serve with beans or rice.

Nutritional Information per Serving:

Calories: 231; Total Fat: 2.5 g; Carbs: 15.9 g; Dietary Fiber: 8.5 g; Sugars: 3.7 g; Protein: 5.9 g; Cholesterol: 0 mg; Sodium: 582 mg

Yummy Brussels Sprouts

Yield: 4 Servings

Total Time: 16 Minutes

Prep Time: 10 Minutes

Cook Time: 6 Minutes

Ingredients

- 2 pound Brussels sprouts, halved
- 1 tbsp. chopped almonds
- 1 tbsp. rice vinegar
- 2 tbsp. sriracha sauce
- 1/4 cup soy sauce
- 2 tbsp. sesame oil
- 1/2 tbsp. cayenne pepper

- 1 tbsp. smoked paprika
- 1 tsp. onion powder
- 2 tsp. garlic powder
- 1 tsp. red pepper flakes
- Salt and pepper

Directions

Set your pot to sauté and add in almond; cook for about 3 minutes and then stir in all the seasonings and liquid ingredients. Stir in Brussels sprouts and set on manual high for 3 minutes. When done, quick release pressure and serve over rice.

Nutritional Information per Serving:

Calories: 185; Total Fat: 8.7 g; Carbs: 24.1 g; Dietary Fiber: 9.8 g; Sugars: 5.8 g; Protein: 8.8 g; Cholesterol: 0 mg; Sodium: 114 mg

Instant Pot Garlicky Mashed Potatoes

Yield: 4 Servings

Total Time: 9 Minutes

Prep Time: 5 Minutes

Cook Time: 4 Minutes

Ingredients

- 6 cloves garlic, chopped
- 1 cup vegetable broth
- 4 Yukon gold potatoes, diced
- 1/2 cup almond milk
- 1/4 cup chopped parsley
- 1/8 tsp. sea salt

Directions

In your instant pot, mix garlic, broth, and potatoes and lock the lid; set to manual for four minutes and then release the pressure naturally. Transfer the potato mixture to a large bowl and mash with a potato masher until smooth.

Add soy milk to your desired consistency and then stir in parsley and salt. Serve hot!

Nutritional Information per Serving:

Calories: 243; Total Fat: 0.8 g; Carbs: 24.7 g; Dietary Fiber: 11.2 g; Sugars: 12 g; Protein: 4.5 g; Cholesterol: 0 mg; Sodium: 415 mg

INSTANT POT WHOLE30 DINNER RECIPES

Instant Pot Beef and Sweet Potato Stew

Yield: 10 Servings

Total Time: 35 Minutes

Prep Time: 10 Minutes

Cook Time: 25 Minutes

Ingredients

- 2 pounds ground beef
- 3 cups beef stock
- 2 sweet potatoes, peeled and diced
- 1 clove garlic, minced
- 1 onion, diced
- 1 (14-oz) can petite minced tomatoes
- 2 (14-oz) cans tomato sauce
- 3-4 tbsp. chili powder

- ¼ tsp. oregano
- 2 tsp. salt
- ½ tsp. black pepper
- Cilantro, optional, for garnish

Directions

Brown the beef in a pan over medium heat; drain excess fat and then transfer it to an instant pot. Stir in the remaining ingredients and lock lid; cook on high for 25 minutes and then release pressure naturally. Garnish with cilantro and serve warm.

Nutritional Information per Serving:

Calories: 240; Total Fat: 6.4 g; Carbs: 15.1 g; Dietary Fiber: 3.5 g; Sugars: 4.2 g; Protein: 30.3 g; Cholesterol: 81 mg; Sodium: 1201 mg

Instant Pot Turkey Chili

Yield: 4-6 Servings

Total Time: 4 Hours 10 Minutes

Prep Time: 10 Minutes

Cook Time: 4 Hours

Ingredients

- 1 1/4 pounds lean ground turkey
- 1 garlic clove, minced
- 1 large red onion, chopped
- 1 (15-oz.) can black beans
- 1 (8-oz.) can tomato sauce
- 1 (28-oz.) can crushed tomatoes
- 1 green bell pepper, chopped
- 1 red bell pepper, chopped
- 1 1/2 cups frozen corn kernels
- 1 package (1 1/4-oz.) chili seasoning mix
- 1/2 tsp. sea salt

Directions

In a large skillet, cook ground turkey, garlic, and onion until turkey is no longer pink; transfer the mixture to your instant pot and stir in the remaining ingredients.

Lock lid and cook on high for 20 minutes. Release pressure naturally and serve hot with your favorite toppings.

Nutritional Information per Serving:

Calories: 495; Total Fat: 8.2 g; Carbs: 70.2 g; Dietary Fiber: 17.6 g; Sugars: 14.9 g; Protein: 39.3 g; Cholesterol: 68 mg; Sodium: 686 mg

Healthy Instant Pot Ground Beef Jalapeno Stew

Yield: 6 Servings

Total Time: 4 Hours 25 Minutes

Prep Time: 25 Minutes

Cook Time: 4 Hours

Ingredients

- 1-1.5 pounds ground beef
- 1 red bell pepper, chopped
- 1 green bell pepper, chopped
- 2 jalapeños, finely diced
- 1 acorn squash, peeled and diced
- 2 zucchinis, sliced
- 4 small carrots, sliced
- 3 green onions, thinly sliced

- 1 (28 ounce) can whole peeled tomatoes
- 4 tbsp. chili powder
- 1 (6 ounce) can tomato paste
- 1 (14 ounce) can tomato sauce

Instructions

Brown ground beef in a pan over medium heat.

In an instant pot, combine the browned beef, bell peppers, Jalapeños, zucchinis, carrots, onions, and squash. Add whole tomatoes and stir with a spatula to mix well. Stir in chili powder along with the remaining ingredients and lock lid; cook on high for 25 minutes. Serve over green salad.

Nutritional Information per Serving:

Calories: 265; Total Fat: 6.1 g; Carbs: 28.4 g; Dietary Fiber: 7.4 g; Sugars: 11.7 g; Protein: 27.9 g; Cholesterol: 68 mg; Sodium: 509 mg

Instant Pot Italian Pulled Pork Ragu

Yield: 10 Servings

Total Time: 1 Hour

Prep Time: 10 Minutes

Cook Time: 50 Minutes

Ingredients:

- 1 pound pork tenderloin
- 1 tsp. kosher salt
- black pepper, to taste
- 1 tsp. olive oil
- 5 cloves garlic, minced
- 4 cups crushed tomatoes
- 1 cup roasted red peppers
- 2 sprigs fresh thyme
- 2 bay leaves
- 1 tbsp. chopped fresh parsley, divided

Directions:

Season the pork with salt and pepper.

Set your instant pot on sauté mode and add oil; sauté garlic for about two minutes until tender and then add pork; brown for about two minutes per side and then stir in the remaining ingredients.

Lock lid and cook on high for 45 minutes. Release the pressure naturally and serve.

Nutrition Information Per Serving:

Calories: 93; Total Fat: 1.5 G; Carbs: 6.5 G; Dietary Fiber: 0 G; Sugars: 3 G; Protein: 11 G; Cholesterol: Sodium: 347 Mg

Jamaican Jerk Pork Roast – Low Carb & Whole 30

Yield: 10 Servings

Total Time: 1 Hour

Prep Time: 10 Minutes

Cook Time: 50 Minutes

Ingredients

- 4 pound pork shoulder
- 1 tbsp. olive oil
- 1/4 cup Jamaican Jerk spice blend
- 1/2 cup beef broth

Directions

Rub the roast with oil and dust with spice blend; set an instant pot on sauté mode and brown roast on both sides; stir in broth and lock lid. Cook on high for 45 minutes and then release pressure naturally.

Shred and serve.

Nutritional Information per Serving:

Calories: 544; Total Fat: 40.3 g; Carbs: 0.1 g; Dietary Fiber: 0 g; Sugars: 0 g; Protein: 42.5 g; Cholesterol: 163 mg; Sodium: 162 mg

Instant Pot Barbacoa

Yield: 8 Servings

Total Time: 1 Hour 10 Minutes

Prep Time: 10 Minutes

Ingredients

- 3 pounds grass-fed chuck roast, diced into large chunks
- 6 garlic cloves
- 1 large onion, chopped
- 2 4oz cans of green chilies
- 3 dried chipotle peppers, chopped
- 3 tbsp. coconut vinegar
- 1 cup fresh lime juice
- 1/2 cup water

- 1 tsp. salt
- 1 tsp. pepper
- 1 tbsp. cumin
- 1 tbsp. oregano

Directions

Combine all ingredients in your instant pot; lock lid and cook on high for 60 minutes. When done, release pressure naturally and shred before serving.

Nutritional Information per Serving:

Calories: 276; Total Fat: 11 g; Carbs: 25.2 g; Dietary Fiber: 9.3 g; Sugars: 13.5 g; Protein: 23.9 g; Cholesterol: 60 mg; Sodium: 421 mg

Pressure Cooker AIP Italian Beef (Paleo, Gluten Free, Instant Pot)

Yield: 8 Servings

Total Time: 1 Hours 40 Minutes

Prep Time: 10 Minutes

Cook Time: 1 Hour 30 Minutes

Ingredients

- 3 pound grass-fed chuck roast
- 6 cloves garlic
- 1 tsp. marjoram
- 1 tsp. basil
- 1 tsp. oregano
- 1/2 tsp. ground ginger
- 1 tsp. onion powder
- 2 tsp. garlic powder
- 1 tsp. salt
- 1/4 cup apple cider vinegar
- 1 cup beef broth

Directions

Cut slits in the roast with a sharp knife and then stuff with garlic cloves.

In a bowl, whisk together marjoram, basil, oregano, ground ginger, onion powder, garlic powder, and salt until well blended; rub the seasoning all over the roast and place it in your instant pot.

Add vinegar and broth and lock lid; cook on high for 90 minutes. Release pressure naturally and then shred meat with a fork.

Serve along with cooking juices.

Nutritional Information per Serving:

Calories: 174; Total Fat: 9.2 g; Carbs: 1.9 g; Dietary Fiber: 0.3 g; Sugars: 0.4 g; Protein: 21 g; Cholesterol: 60 mg; Sodium: 487 mg

Healthy Quinoa Bowl with Grilled Steak & Veggies

Yield: 4 Servings

Total Time: 30 Minutes

Prep Time: 10 Minutes

Cook Time: 20 Minutes

Ingredients

- 2 cups quinoa
- 16 ounces steak, cut into bite-size pieces
- 1 cup baby arugula

- 1 cup sweet potato slices
- 1 cup red pepper, chopped
- 1 cup scallions, chopped
- 1/2 cup toasted salted pepitas
- 2 tsp. fresh cilantro leaves
- 2 cups microgreens
- 2 tbsp. tomato sauce
- 2 tbsp. extra-virgin olive oil
- Kosher salt
- Black pepper
- 1 tbsp. fresh lime juice

Directions

Cook quinoa in your instant pot, as described in breakfast recipes.

Meanwhile, grill steak to medium rare for about 15 minutes. Grill scallions, red pepper, and sweet potatoes along with the steak until tender.

Place cooked quinoa in a bowl; top with grilled steak, scallions, veggies, pepitas, cilantro, and microgreens.

In a small bowl, whisk together oil, tomato sauce, salt, and pepper until well blended; drizzle over the steak mixture and serve drizzled with lime juice.

Nutritional Information per Serving:

Calories: 527; Total Fat: 17 g; Carbs: 48.8 g; Dietary Fiber: 6.4 g; Sugars: 2.4; Protein: 45 g; Cholesterol: 82 mg; Sodium: 24 mg

Asparagus Quinoa & Steak Bowl

Yield: 4 Servings

Total Time: 25 Minutes

Prep Time: 10

Cook Time: 15 Minutes

Ingredients

- 1-1/2 cups white quinoa
- Olive oil cooking spray
- 3/4 pound beef top sirloin steak, diced
- 1/2 tsp. low-sodium steak seasoning
- 1/2 cup chopped red bell pepper
- 1/2 cup chopped red onion
- 1 cup frozen asparagus cuts
- 2 ½ tbsp. tamari sauce

Directions

Cook quinoa in your instant pot, as described in breakfast recipes.

In the meantime, coat a large skillet with cooking spray and heat over medium high heat.

Sprinkle beef with the steak seasoning and cook in the skillet for about three minutes; add bell pepper and red onion and cook for three minutes more or until beef is browned. Add asparagus and continue cooking for four minutes or until asparagus is heated through.

Stir tamari sauce into the quinoa until well combined and toss it with the beef mixture before serving.

Nutritional Information per Serving:

Calories: 345; Total Fat: 7.9 g; Carbs: 32.8; Dietary Fiber: 4.2 g; Sugars: 2 g; Protein: 32.9 g; Cholesterol: 76 mg; Sodium: 60 mg

Instant Pot Lemon Olive Chicken

Yield: 4 Servings

Total Time: 30 Minutes

Prep Time: 10 Minutes

Cook Time: 20 Minutes

Ingredients

- 4 boneless skinless chicken breasts
- ½ cup coconut oil
- ¼ tsp. black pepper
- ½ tsp. cumin
- 1 tsp. sea salt
- 1 cup chicken bone broth

- 2 tbsp. fresh lemon juice
- ½ cup red onion, sliced
- 1 can pitted green olives
- 1/2 lemon, thinly sliced

Directions

Generously season chicken breasts with cumin, pepper and salt; set your instant pot on sauté mode and heat the coconut oil; add chicken and brown both sides. Stir in the remaining ingredients; bring to a gentle simmer and then lock lid.

Cook on high for 10 minutes and then use quick release method to release pressure.

Nutritional Information per Serving:

Calories: 420; Total Fat: 38.7 g; Carbs: 0.6 g; Dietary Fiber: 0.2 g; Sugars: 0.2 g; Protein: 42.4 g; Cholesterol: 130 mg; Sodium: 662 mg

Instant Pot Chicken Shawarma

Yield: 8 Servings

Total Time: 25 Minutes

Prep Time: 10 Minutes

Cook Time: 15 Minutes

Ingredients

- 1 pound chicken thighs
- 1 pound chicken breasts, sliced
- 1/8 tsp. cinnamon
- 1/4 tsp. chili powder
- 1 tsp. ground cumin
- 1/4 tsp. ground allspice
- 1/4 tsp. granulated garlic
- 1/2 tsp. turmeric
- 1 tsp. paprika
- Pinch of salt
- Pinch of pepper
- 1 cup chicken broth

Directions

Mix all ingredients in your instant pot and lock lid; cook on poultry setting for 15 minutes and then release pressure naturally.

Serve chicken with sauce over mashed sweet potato drizzled with tahini sauce.

Nutritional Information per Serving:

Calories: 223; Total Fat: 8.7 g; Carbs: 0.7 g; Dietary Fiber: 0.2 g; Sugars: 0.2 g; Protein: 35.5 g; Cholesterol: 101 mg; Sodium: 214 mg

Instant Pot Chipotle Shredded Beef

Yield: 8 Servings

Total Time: 1 Hour 30 Minutes

Prep Time: 20 Minutes

Cook Time: 1 Hour 10 Minutes

Ingredients

- 2 tbsp. olive oil
- 3 pounds beef chuck roast
- 1 tbsp. adobo sauce
- 1 chipotle in adobo, chopped
- ½ tsp. chili powder
- 2 tsp. dried oregano
- 2 tsp. dried cumin
- 1 tsp. black pepper
- 2 tsp. salt

- 1 cup fresh cilantro, chopped
- 1 green bell pepper, diced
- 1 onion, chopped
- 1 cup water

Directions

Generously season the roast with salt and pepper.

Add olive oil to your instant pot and press the sauté button; add the roast and brown on both sides; spread adobo sauce and chipotle pepper over the roast and sprinkle with seasoning and cilantro; add bell pepper and onions and pour water around the edges of meat. Lock lid; cook on high for 60 minutes and then release pressure naturally.

Shred meat and serve with cooking sauce.

Nutritional Information per Serving:

Calories: 665; Total Fat: 51.1 g; Carbs: 3.8 g; Dietary Fiber: 0.9 g; Sugars: 1.9 g; Protein: 45 g; Cholesterol: 175 mg; Sodium: 756 mg

Delicious Instant Pot Seafood Stew

Yield: 6 Servings

Total Time: 35 Minutes

Prep Time: 15 Minutes

Cook Time: 20 Minutes

Ingredients:

- 2 pounds seafood (1 pound large shrimp & 1 pound scallops)
- 1/2 cup chopped white onion
- 3 garlic cloves, minced
- 1 tbsp. tomato paste
- 1 can (28 oz.) crushed tomatoes
- 4 cups vegetable broth
- 1 pound yellow potatoes, diced
- 1 tsp. dried basil
- 1 tsp. dried thyme
- 1 tsp. dried oregano
- 1/8 tsp. cayenne pepper
- 1/4 tsp. crush red pepper flakes
- 1/2 tsp. celery salt
- salt and pepper
- handful of chopped parsley

Directions:

Mix all ingredients, except seafood, in your instant pot and lock lid; cook on high for about 15 minutes. Quick release the pressure and then stir in seafood and continue; lock lid and cook on high for five minutes and then let pressure come down on its own. Serve hot with crusty gluten-free bread and garnished with parsley.

Nutritional Information per Serving:

Calories: 323; Total Fat: 5.3 g; Carbs: 7.7 g; Dietary Fiber: 0.8 g; Sugars: 1.9 g; Protein: 57.1 g; Cholesterol: 478 mg; Sodium: 1323 mg

Instant Pot Coconut Curry Shrimp

Yield: 4 Servings

Total Time: 20 Minutes

Prep Time: 5 Minutes

Cook Time: 15 Hours

Ingredients

- 1 pound shelled shrimp
- 15 ounces water
- 4 cups coconut milk
- ½ cup Thai red curry sauce

- ¼ cup cilantro
- 2½ tsp. garlic-lemon seasoning

Directions

In your instant pot, combine water, coconut milk, red curry paste, cilantro, and lemon garlic seasoning; stir to mix well and lock lid; cook on high for 10 minutes and then release the pressure quickly. Add shrimp and continue cooking for another five minutes and then release pressure naturally.

Serve garnished with cilantro.

Nutritional Information per Serving:

Calories: 624; Total Fat: 52.6 g; Carbs: 13.5 g; Dietary Fiber: 4.7 g; Sugars: 7.1 g; Protein: 30.7 g; Cholesterol: 239 mg; Sodium: 312 mg

Slow Cooker Thai Seafood Boil

Yield: 4 Servings

Total Time: 4 Hours 10 Minutes

Prep Time: 10 Minutes

Cook Time: 4 Hours

Ingredients

- ½ pound snow crab
- ½ pound shrimp (in shells)
- 1 stalk lemongrass, outer layer and top inch removed
- 2 tsp. ginger
- ¼ cup of fresh mint, chopped
- 1 lime, cut in half
- 2 garlic cloves, minced
- 1 small onion, cut into quarters
- 2 cups coconut milk
- 32 ounces homemade broth
- ½ tsp. cumin
- 1 tsp. salt
- 1 celery stalk, cut into 1-inch pieces
- 1 pound sweet potatoes, cut into quarters
- 1 bell pepper, cut into 1-inch pieces
- 1 ear of sweet corn, cut into 3-inch chunks

Directions

Crush the end of the lemongrass stalk with a rolling pin until soft; transfer to an instant pot along with ginger, mint, lime, garlic, onion, coconut milk, broth, cumin, and salt. Stir to combine well and then add in celery and sweet potatoes. Lock lid and cook on high for 10 minutes. Quick release pressure and then add corn, bell pepper, and seafood; lock lid and continue cooking for 10 minutes. Release pressure naturally.

Strain the liquid and serve.

Nutritional Information per Serving:

Calories: 595; Total Fat: 31.5 g; Carbs: 52.6 g; Dietary Fiber: 9.4 g; Sugars: 4.7 g; Protein: 17.7 g; Cholesterol: 176 mg; Sodium: 918 mg

Hot Lemony Instant Pot Tilapia with Asparagus

Yield: 6 Servings

Total Time: 2 Hours 15 Minutes

Prep Time: 15 Minutes

Cook Time: 2 Hours

Ingredients

- 6 tilapia filets
- 1 bundle of asparagus
- 12 tbsp. lemon juice
- Lemon pepper seasoning
- 3 tbsp. melted coconut oil

Directions

Divide asparagus into equal amounts per each fillet.

Place each fillet in the center of a piece of foil and sprinkle with about 1 tsp. lemon pepper seasoning; drizzle with about 2 tbsp. lemon juice and about ½ tbsp. melted coconut oil. Top each filet with the asparagus and fold the foil to form a packet. Repeat with the remaining ingredients and then place the packets into an instant pot. Lock lid and cook on high for 15 minutes.

Nutritional Information per Serving:

Calories: 181; Total Fat: 11.5 g; Carbs: 1.8 g; Dietary Fiber: 0.7 g; Sugars: 1.3 g; Protein: 27.3 g; Cholesterol: 60 mg; Sodium: 404 mg

Instant Pot Citrus Tilapia

Yield: 4 Servings

Total Time: 2 Hours 10 Minutes

Prep Time: 10 Minutes

Cook Time: 2 Hours

Ingredients

- 4 tilapia filets
- 1 10-ounce can mandarin oranges
- 2 tbsp. minced garlic
- 2 tbsp. coconut oil
- Sea salt and pepper

Directions

Arrange fish side by side on a large piece of aluminum foil and sprinkle with garlic and coconut oil evenly. Top the fish with oranges and season with salt and pepper; fold the foil to wrap the content well.

Place in an instant pot and lock lid; cook on high for 15 minutes.

Nutritional Information per Serving:

Calories: 201; Total Fat: 9.3 g; Carbs: 8.2 g; Dietary Fiber: 0.6 g; Sugars: 6.3 g; Protein: 22.7 g; Cholesterol: 50 mg; Sodium: 334 mg

INSTANT POT WHOLE30 DESSERTS AND SNACKS

Power Protein Stuffed Strawberries

Yield: 4 Servings

Total Time: 25 Minutes

Prep Time: 15 Minutes

Cook Time: 10 Minutes

Ingredients

- 24 strawberries
- 1 ripe banana
- ¼ cup quinoa, uncooked
- 12 almonds, chopped
- ½ tsp. cinnamon

- ½ tsp. almond extract
- 1 tsp. cocoa powder, unsweetened
- ½ tbsp. raw honey

Directions

Cook the quinoa in your instant pot; see recipe in breakfast section.

Now, combine the cooked quinoa, banana, cocoa powder, cinnamon, honey, and almond extract in a large bowl and mix well; then, set aside to cool.

Rinse the berries with water and gently pat them dry. Use a paring knife, preferably a small one, to remove the tops and to also scoop out some of the flesh of each berry.

You can combine the scooped-out flesh with the quinoa mixture if so desired then scoop this mixture into the center of each berry. Finally top with the almonds and chill in the fridge for an hour or two before serving. Enjoy!

Nutritional Information per Serving:

Calories: 476; Total Fat: 11.3 g; Carbs: 88.4 g; Dietary Fiber: 14.8 g; Sugars: 35.4 g; Protein: 12.7 g; Cholesterol: 0 mg; Sodium: 8 mg

Avocado Brownies

Yield: 8 Brownies
Total Time: 30 Minutes
Prep Time: 5 Minutes
Cook Time: 25 Minutes

Ingredients

- 1 cup chopped chocolate
- 2 ripe avocados
- 1 tsp. raw honey
- 2 tsp. vanilla extract
- 4 eggs
- 1 cup ground almonds
- ½ cup cocoa powder
- ¼ tsp. salt

Directions

Prepare an 8-inch baking pan by lining it with foil and then coating with non-stick cooking spray.

Add chocolate to a bowl and place over a large saucepan of boiling water. Stir until chocolate is melted. Remove from heat and let cool.

Meanwhile, prepare the batter: in a bowl, mash the avocados; add honey and stir to combine. Whisk in vanilla extract and eggs until well blended. Gradually whisk in the chocolate until well incorporated. Stir in ground almonds, cocoa powder, and salt until well blended.

Transfer the batter to the prepared baking pan and cover with a paper towel and then with aluminum foil. Place the pan on a trivet. Add water to your instant pot and carefully place the trivet in the pot and lock lid. Press "cake" button and then set mode to "less." Adjust cooking time to 50 minutes and when done, release pressure naturally. Let cool completely before cutting into squares. These brownies are best served chilled.

Nutritional Information per Serving:

Calories: 330; Total Fat: 24.9 g; Carbs: 22.6 g; Dietary Fiber: 7.2 g; Sugars: 12 g; Protein: 8.8 g; Cholesterol: 87 mg; Sodium: 125 mg

Instant Pot Blood Orange Marmalade

Yield: 2 Servings

Total Time: 17 Minutes

Prep Time: 5 Minutes

Cook Time: 12 Minutes

Ingredients

- 4 whole blood oranges, quartered and thinly sliced
- ½ cup fresh lemon juice
- 2 tbsp. raw honey

Directions

Place the oranges, along with their juice, and the lemon juice in your instant pot and add a cup of water; lock lid and cook on manual for 12 minutes. When done, press cancel button and let pressure come down on its own. Stir in honey and press the sauté button; cook, stirring constantly, until the thermometer reads 105°F.

Strain your marmalade through a fine mesh into a jar and seal with lid; chill in the fridge before serving.

Nutritional Information per Serving:

Calories: 251; Total Fat: 0.9 g; Carbs: 61.8 g; Dietary Fiber: 9.1 g; Sugars: 52.9 g; Protein: 4 g; Cholesterol: 0 mg; Sodium: 13 mg

Instant Pot Cheesecake

Yield: Makes 1 cake, 8 to 12 slices

Total Time: 40 Minutes

Prep Time: 20 Minutes

Cook Time: 20 Minutes

Ingredients

Crust

- ½ cup dates, chopped, soaked in water for at least 15 min., soaking liquid reserved
- ½ cup walnuts
- 1 cup quick oats

Filling

- ½ cup vanilla almond milk
- ¼ cup coconut palm sugar
- ½ cup coconut flour
- 1 cup cashews, soaked in water for at least 2 hours
- 1 tsp. vanilla extract
- 2 tbsp. lemon juice
- 1 to 2 tsp. grated lemon zest
- ½ cup fresh berries or 6 figs, sliced
- 1 tbsp. arrowroot powder

Directions

Pour 1 ½ cups of water into an instant pot and insert a rack.

Make the crust: in a food processor, process together all the crust ingredients until smooth and press the mixture into the bottom of a springform pan.

Make the filling: add cashews along with soaking liquid to a blender and process until very smooth; add milk, palm sugar, coconut flour, lemon juice, lemon zest, and vanilla and blend until well combined; add arrowroot and continue blending until mixed and pour into the crust. Smooth the top and cover the springform pan with foil. Place the pan into the pot and lock lid; cook on high pressure for 20 minutes and then let pressure come down naturally.

Carefully remove the pan from the pot and remove the foil; let the cake cool completely and top with fruit to serve.

Nutritional Information per Serving:

Calories: 252; Total Fat: 13.6 g; Carbs: 29.4 g; Dietary Fiber: 3.4 g; Sugars: 12.8 g; Protein: 6.4 g; Cholesterol: 0 mg; Sodium: 29 mg

Instant Pot Dulce de Leche

Yield: 6 Servings

Total Time: 55 Minutes

Prep Time: 5 Minutes

Cook Time: 50 Minutes

Ingredients:

- 2 (14-ounce) cans sweetened coconut cream

Directions:

Add coconut cream to a canning jar and secure with lid; place a steamer basket in your instant pot and add the jar with coconut cream. Lock the lid and cook on high pressure for 50 minutes. When done, release pressure naturally. Remove the jar and let the dulce de leche cool before stirring. Enjoy!

Nutritional Information per Serving:

Calories: 614; Total Fat: 28.3 g; Carbs: 85.1 g; Dietary Fiber: 0 g; Sugars: 42.5 g; Protein: 4.8 g; Cholesterol: 0 mg; Sodium: 286 mg

Ratatouille Riviera-Style

Yield: 4 Servings

Total Time: 35 Minutes

Prep Time: 15 Minutes

Cook Time: 20 Minutes

Ingredients:

- 1 tbsp. extra-virgin olive oil
- 3 cloves garlic, minced
- 2 onions, chopped
- 500g eggplant, chopped
- 400g squash, diced
- 4 tomatoes, chopped
- 2 tsp. dried basil
- 1 red capsicum, chopped
- 1 green capsicum, chopped
- ½ tsp. ground pepper
- ½ tsp. dried thyme
- 1 tsp. salt

Directions

Sauté garlic and onion in your instant pot until softened and fragrant; stir in all veggies, except tomatoes, and cook for a few minutes until tender. Add in the tomatoes and lock lid; cook on high pressure for five minutes and then let pressure come down on its own. Serve.

Nutritional Information per Serving:

Calories: 126; Total Fat: 4.3 g; Carbs: 21.6 g; Dietary Fiber: 8.4 g; Sugars: 11.1 g; Protein: 4.3 g; Cholesterol: 0 mg; Sodium: 603 mg

Lemon Broccoli

Yield: 4-6 Servings

Total Time: 7 Minutes

Prep Time: 5 Minutes

Cook Time: 2 Minutes

Ingredients:

- 1 cup water
- 900 g broccoli, tough parts removed and ends scored
- 4 tbsp. lemon juice
- salt and pepper

Directions

Add the water to your instant pot and add in broccoli; drizzle with lemon juice and season with salt and pepper. Lock lid and cook on high for two minutes and then release pressure naturally. Serve.

Nutritional Information per Serving:

Calories: 126; Total Fat: 4.3 g; Carbs: 21.6 g; Dietary Fiber: 8.4 g; Sugars: 11.1 g; Protein: 4.3 g; Cholesterol: 0 mg; Sodium: 603 mg

Instant Pot Baked Potatoes

Yield: 4 Servings

Total Time: 25 Minutes

Prep Time: 5 Minutes

Cook Time: 20 Minutes

Ingredients

- 2 pounds medium potatoes
- 1 cup water

Directions

Add the potatoes to your instant pot and poke each potato, facing up, with a knife several times; add water and lock the lid. Cook on high pressure for 10 minutes and then release pressure naturally.

Transfer the potatoes onto an oven rack and bake for about 15 minutes or until crispy, but fluffy.

Nutritional Information per Serving:

Calories: 156; Total Fat: 0.2 g; Carbs: 35.6 g; Dietary Fiber: 5.4 g; Sugars: 2.6 g; Protein: 3.8 g; Cholesterol: 0 mg; Sodium: 15 mg

Strawberry-Rhubarb Compote w/ Fresh Mint

Yield: 4 Cups

Total Time: 40 Minutes

Prep Time: 10 Minutes

Cook Time: 30 Minutes

Ingredients

- 2 pound rhubarb, peeled and chopped
- 1 pound strawberries, stemmed and quartered
- ⅓ cup water
- 3 tbsp. raw honey
- Fresh mint, minced

Directions

Combine rhubarb and water in your instant pot and lock the lid; press manual and set to 10 minutes.

When done, let pressure come down on its own and then stir in strawberries and honey; close the lid and let simmer for about 20 minutes. Serve hot garnished with fresh mint.

Nutritional Information per Serving:

Calories: 118; Total Fat: 0.8 g; Carbs: 28 g; Dietary Fiber: 6.4 g; Sugars: 17.1 g; Protein: 2.8 g; Cholesterol: 0 mg; Sodium: 11 mg

Parting Shot…

Thank you for downloading this book!

I hope this whole30 recipe guide has helped you learn that a whole food diet can be very tasty and, most of all, why the diet is just what you need to steer your health in the right direction.

The next step is to jump right into the diet by making healthy and smart whole food choices to ensure you meet your recommended daily nutrition. If you are starting out on whole30 diet, you should join an online whole30 diet group that will further guide you on the best way to take up the diet and tips and tricks to stay on it.

We have seen the immense health benefits of the whole food diet. Combine it with regular exercise, clean water, and healthy habits and you will discover the fountain of health and youth.

Now, get your apron ready and start cooking these yummy dishes that will bring back food to soul of your home. All the best!

Made in the USA
Middletown, DE
27 December 2017